ABOUT THE PROSTATE

Understanding Prostate Health: Anatomy, Functions, and Common Concerns

BY

DR. JAMES K. WEISS

TABLE OF CONTENTS

Introduction

I'm here to shed light on the complex process that leads to the development of prostate cancer. Understanding the causes of prostate cancer, a common ailment in males can enable us to take proactive steps for early identification and prevention. Men's total health is contingent upon maintaining a healthy prostate. The small, walnut-shaped prostate glands in men are located beneath the bladder. By producing and secreting chemicals that support and protect sperm, it plays a critical part in the male reproductive system. The prostate gland's health refers to its state, which includes its size, functionality, and lack of disease.

Any sickness or disorder that affects the prostate gland, a little gland in males that is situated below the rectum and beneath the bladder, is referred to as prostate disease. An essential component of the male reproductive system, the prostate gland secretes a fluid that aids in nourishing and transporting sperm during ejaculation.

Prostate disease refers to a broad variety of disorders, from relatively minor and readily curable problems like prostatitis (prostate gland inflammation) to more serious problems like prostate cancer.A number of common conditions, including prostatitis, benign prostatic hyperplasia (BPH), and prostate cancer, can have an effect on the prostate. These problems could result in pain, suffering, or even serious health problems. Men of all ages must therefore comprehend the fundamentals of prostate health and how to preserve it. The following parts will cover the anatomy and physiology of the prostate, prevalent disorders that might affect it, risk factors for prostate problems, and the necessity of routine prostate exams. We'll also cover lifestyle modifications men can adopt to better the condition of their prostates. Healthy prostate cells undergo a shift that causes them to proliferate uncontrollably and form a tumor, which is how cancer develops. A tumor may be benign or malignant. Malignant refers to the ability of a cancerous tumor to develop and metastasize to different body regions. If a tumor is benign, it can enlarge but won't spread.

Comparing prostate cancer to other cancers, it is a little different. This is due to the fact that many prostate cancers do not readily spread to other body areas. Some forms of prostate cancer grow very slowly and may go years or even decades without showing any signs or issues. Even when prostate cancer has spread to other bodily areas, it is frequently treatable for a very long time. Therefore, men with prostate cancer, even those with advanced disease, may have a long lifespan of good health and quality of life. However, if the cancer cannot be effectively treated with current therapies, it might result in symptoms including discomfort and weariness as well as occasionally cause death. Monitoring growth over time to determine whether it is expanding slowly or quickly is a crucial component of controlling prostate cancer. When prostate cancer in its early stages is discovered, it may be treated or put on surveillance (close observation). Although advanced prostate cancer is not "curable," there are several effective treatments available. Treatment can halt the spread of advanced prostate cancer.

Men's general health, specifically prostate health, is crucial. Despite this, many men disregard and undervalue the condition of their prostates. However, improving your prostate health should be one of your top goals if you're a male.

Chapter 1

What is Prostate:

Men and those who were assigned male at birth (AMAB) have a tiny gland called the prostate that is located in front of the rectum and beneath the bladder. It is made up of glandular tissues and connective tissues. Its muscles aid in pushing semen through your urethra and it adds fluid to semen. Prostate cancer, prostatitis, and benign prostatic hyperplasia (BPH) are all conditions that can affect your prostate.

The prostate may be a secretor located in front of the body portion, beneath the bladder. It is essential to the portion of the male genitalia that generates spermatozoan-carrying fluids.

The following people have Prostate

- Men
- Trans-women
- Non-binary people who were assigned male at birth

- Some intersex people

Where is the prostate located?

Your urethra, which is the tube that takes pee out of the body, is surrounded by your prostate, which is located below your bladder and in front of your rectum. The middle of your prostate is where your urethra is located.

What does a prostate do for a man?

Your semen (ejaculate) contains extra fluid from your prostate. When you orgasm, a whitish-gray fluid called ejaculate comes out of your penis.
Citric acid, zinc, and enzymes found in the fluid lubricate your urethra and nourish sperm cells. Your body's urethra is a conduit via which urine and ejaculate exit.
Semen fluid, which contains sperm made in the testicles, is produced by it. It prevents urine from being included during ejaculation.

What does the prostate look like?

Your prostate has five lobes: anterior (in the front) and posterior (in the back) lobes, two lateral lobes (on the sides) and one median (in the middle) lobe. Connective tissues and glandular tissues make up its structure. The prostatic fascia covers your prostate. Prostatic fascia is a sheet of stretchy connective tissue.
If it gets too big, your prostate can block pee from passing through the urethra and out the penis.

How big is the prostate?

Your prostate is about the size of a walnut.
The prostate usually gets larger after age 40 (benign prostatic hyperplasia). It can grow from the size of a walnut to the size of a lemon. Benign prostatic hyperplasia (BPH) isn't cancerous, and it doesn't increase your risk of developing prostate cancer.

Your prostate weighs about 1 ounce (30 grams), which is as heavy as five U.S. quarters.

What are the common conditions and disorders that affect the prostate?

Prostate pain is a medical condition characterized by pain, discomfort, or inflammation in the prostate gland. It is a common condition that affects men of all ages, and it can range from mild to severe. Prostate pain can occur due to various reasons, including infections, inflammation, or prostate cancer.

The common conditions that affect your prostate include:

Prostate cancer

Men and people who were assigned male at birth (AMAB) are more likely to get prostate cancer than any other type of cancer.

Inflammation (prostatitis)

Acute bacterial prostatitis, chronic bacterial prostatitis, chronic pelvic pain syndrome (CPPS), and asymptomatic inflammatory prostatitis are the four forms of prostatitis that can inflame your prostate gland.

In males and people AMAB under 50, it is the most prevalent urinary tract problem, while in men and AMAB over 50, it is the third most prevalent.

Prostate inflammation refers to inflammation of the prostate gland itself. Men can be significantly impacted by the illness. Pain, particularly in the perineal region and during urination, is a sign that the prostate is inflamed.

Benign prostatic hyperplasia

Your prostate can grow as a result of BPH, which could result in urethral obstructions. As people get older, the prostate enlarges to some extent in almost all men and AMAB.

Chapter 2

What is inflammation of the prostate?

The term "prostatitis" describes the inflammation of the prostate gland, a little organ with a walnut-like form that is located below the bladder and close to the urethra. Men are more susceptible to the illness. It is possible to tell if the prostate is inflamed by its pain, especially in the perineal region and when peeing. Prostatitis is another name for prostatitis in medical terminology, as is the more contemporary phrase prostatitis syndrome.

Bacteria, particularly intestinal bacteria, are frequently involved in cases of prostate inflammation. Through the urinary system or, less frequently, through the blood, the bacteria enter the prostate, where they cause inflammation. However, doctors frequently are unable to identify the origin of the prostatitis. The medical name for when a trigger cannot be found is idiopathic prostatitis.

Prostatitis and the causes are different

Prostate inflammation can take many various forms, each with a unique reason. There are times when bacteria are present and times when no bacterial pathogens are found. Inflammation, which typically results in severe discomfort, is a feature of all forms of prostatitis. Acute and chronic forms can also be recognized; in the latter, the prostate inflammation persists for a protracted period of time.

Based on its underlying causes and clinical presentation, this disorder can affect males of any age and is divided into distinct categories.

Acute and chronic prostatitis (ABP) and causes

In five to ten percent of men with acute prostatitis, the inflammation is brought on by a bacterial infection. The germs often enter the prostate gland through the blood and exit through the urinary tract (bladder, urethra). Pathogens trigger tissue inflammation there.

Escherichia coli (E. coli) and Enterococcus faecalis are the most frequent gut bacteria associated with prostate inflammation.

There are additional "culprit" microorganisms that could be the reason:

- Other intestinal bacteria
- enterococci
- Klebsiella
- sometimes Pseudomonas aeruginosa

Bacteria that cause sexually transmitted diseases (STDs), such as Chlamydia, Trichomonas, or Neisseria gonorrhoeae (the cause of gonorrhea), may also be involved.

Chronic bacterial prostatic inflammation can eventually result from acute prostatitis. If the inflammation hasn't gone down after three months, this is the case. The chronic type, however, has milder symptoms, such as less pain when urinating.

This is comparable to Chronic Bacterial Prostate (CBP), in which the prostate is chronically inflamed due to recurrent bacterial infections. Although they could be milder and last longer, ABP-like symptoms are present.

Chronic Prostate or Chronic Pelvic Pain Syndrome (CP/CPPS) and causes

Bacteria cannot be detected in the urine or ejaculate in cases with persistent pelvic pain syndrome. Consequently, another name for this condition is chronic abacterial prostatitis. But other types of bacteria might possibly be involved that can't be found in a lab.

Bacteria cannot be detected in the urine or ejaculate in cases with persistent pelvic pain syndrome. Consequently, another name for this condition is chronic abacterial prostatitis. But other types of bacteria might possibly be involved that can't be found in a lab.

illnesses of the central nervous system (CNS), such as bladder emptying disorders

Prostatic efferent ducts becoming smaller due to tumors or stones in the prostate

Urine entering the prostate's ducts can result in prostatic reflux, which can lead to irritation or stone formation.

Narrowing of the urethra, for instance as a result of benign prostatic enlargement

Researchers are talking more and more about psychological factors, but there is still no evidence to support them.

Asymptomatic prostatitis and causes

When a man has silent prostate inflammation, medical professionals can detect inflammation in the blood but cannot detect any symptoms in the patient. He doesn't have any pain, for instance, that might have prompted him to visit a doctor. During a normal exam, doctors commonly discover this type of prostatitis by mistake.

Inflammation of the prostate and the risk factors?

There are other known additional considerations. They raise the possibility of prostate irritation. Among them are, among others:

- Existing underlying disorders, such as diabetes mellitus. Sometimes, high urine sugar levels offer the perfect conditions for bacterial growth. Prostatitis risk is also increased by HIV/AIDS. Previous inflammation of the prostate - prostatitis can come back several times.

- Pelvic injuries from activities like riding a bicycle or a horse can result in either bladder or urethritis, which have separate origins, although germs are frequently involved.

- Bladder catheter: Bacteria can congregate there and travel down the urinary tract to the prostate. Even minor wounds from the catheter are more easily infected by bacteria. Many times, such as after prostate surgery, a temporary bladder catheter is required.

- Immune system impairment, such as after immunosuppressant use following organ transplantation; • prior prostate biopsy, such as when prostate cancer is suspected;

- Prostate inflammation: Painful symptoms are typically present

- Whether prostate inflammation is acute or persistent affects the symptoms. The symptoms of the acute form of prostatitis are typically less severe.

Acute prostatitis and symptoms

Acute prostatitis frequently develops suddenly and without prior notice. Pain is usually how it shows itself. Men with prostatitis also frequently experience severe pain.

The main symptoms are:

- Burning and stinging pain when urinating
- Dribbling and late-onset urinary incontinence
- Weak, thin urine flow - The prostate, which surrounds the urethra, has swelled and is compressing the urethra, which results in this constant urge to urinate because the bladder is not emptying enough
- Frequent bathroom visits, especially at night.

- Pain during bowel motions; discomfort in the bladder, perineum, anus, back, and groin; blood in the urine or semen; and discomfort in the penis or testicles.
- A general and intense feeling of illness;
- Pain during and after ejaculation.
- Symptoms of the flu, such as fever or chills

Urinary retention is a serious complication. Urinary retention can harm the kidneys, so it needs to be treated right away at a clinic.

These symptoms do not all appear in all men with acute prostatitis, nor do they all manifest to the same degree. Each individual experiences different symptoms. However, if you develop such symptoms, visit your doctor or a urology clinic right away. Some unpleasant effects might result from prostate inflammation.

Chronic prostatitis and symptoms

Generally speaking, the symptoms of chronic prostatitis are less severe (rarely accompanied by fever or chills).

- Pressure sensation in the lower abdomen, back, and perineum
- Brown urine and semen, which indicate the presence of blood.
- Recurrent urinary tract infections, a mild urge to urinate more frequently than usual, difficulty emptying the bladder, a loss of desire, and erectile dysfunction brought on by pain during or after ejaculation are all signs of chronic pelvic pain syndrome.

Similar symptoms to those of chronic prostatitis are displayed by chronic pelvic pain syndrome. Men with silent prostatic inflammation do not exhibit any symptoms, as the name suggests.

Tactile Examination

During a palpation exam (also known as a digital rectal exam, or DRE), the doctor places a finger over the rectum and feels the prostate. This is how you may estimate the prostate's size.

The prostate gland is swollen and hence larger than usual when the prostate is inflamed. Additionally, if light pressure is applied to an inflamed prostate, it will hurt intensely.

The fingertip can also cause other prostatic problems.

Urine Test

Elevated leukocyte levels are indicators of inflammation, and doctors employ the so-called "four-vessel test" to identify bacteria (often E. coli) as the source of prostate inflammation. This test identifies the microorganisms that live in each region of the urinary system. The affected man offers four distinct urine samples.

Chapter 3

Prostate Enlargement (Benign Prostatic Hyperplasia)

Benign prostatic hyperplasia (BPH), often known as prostate enlargement, is a prevalent disorder that affects many older men. It involves the prostate gland non-cancerous development, which causes it to enlarge. This growth may cause a number of uncomfortable urinary symptoms. Here, we will delve into the causes, signs, symptoms, diagnosis, and available treatments for BPH.

Composed of glandular tissue, which goes through two primary growth stages—the first of which begins during puberty and doubles in size—and the second of which starts around age 25 and lasts for the majority of an individual's lifetime, BPH typically develops later in the second growth stage, between the ages of 50 and 60.

What is benign prostatic hyperplasia?

BPH, also known as benign prostatic hyperplasia, is a disorder in which men's prostate glands expand but are not malignant. Other names for benign prostatic hyperplasia are benign prostatic blockage and benign prostatic hypertrophy.

As a man ages, the prostate experiences two major growth phases. The prostate increases in size during the initial phase of puberty. Around the age of 25, the second stage of growth starts, and it lasts for the majority of a man's life. The second growth phase frequently coincides with benign prostatic hyperplasia.

The urethra is pinched and pressed against the prostate as it grows in size. A thickening of the bladder wall occurs. The bladder may eventually deteriorate and lose its capacity to empty entirely, leaving some pee in the bladder. The majority of the issues related to benign prostatic hyperplasia are brought on by the constriction of the urethra and urine retention, or the inability to completely empty the bladder.

What causes benign prostatic hyperplasia?

Benign prostatic hyperplasia primarily affects elderly men, but its exact cause is unknown. Men with removed testicles prior to adolescence do not develop benign prostatic hyperplasia. For this reason, some experts think that age and testicular factors may contribute to benign prostatic hyperplasia.

Men create little amounts of estrogen, a female hormone, and testosterone, a masculine hormone, throughout their lives. Men's blood levels of active testosterone decline with age, leaving a higher percentage of estrogen. According to scientific research, benign prostatic hyperplasia may happen because the prostate's greater estrogen content stimulates the function of molecules that encourage prostate cell proliferation.

Another notion revolves around dihydrotestosterone (DHT), a male hormone involved in prostate development and growth. According to several studies, even as blood testosterone levels fall, older men continue to manufacture and accumulate significant levels of DHT in the prostate. This DHT buildup may drive prostate cells to proliferate further. Men who do not make DHT do not get benign prostatic hyperplasia, according to researchers.

How common is benign prostatic hyperplasia?

The most prevalent prostate condition in males over the age of 50 is benign prostatic hyperplasia.

In 2010, up to 14 million men in the United States experienced lower urinary tract symptoms suggestive with benign prostatic hyperplasia.1 Although symptoms of benign prostatic hyperplasia are uncommon before reaching the age of 40, their prevalence and severity increase with age. Benign prostatic hyperplasia affects approximately 50% of men between the ages of 51 and 60, and up to 90% of men over the age of 80.

Who is more likely to develop benign prostatic hyperplasia?

Men who have the following risk factors for benign prostatic hyperplasia:

- age 40 and older
- family history of benign prostatic hyperplasia
- obesity, heart and vascular illness, and type 2 diabetes
- lack of physical activity
- erectile dysfunction

What are the symptoms of benign prostatic hyperplasia?

Lower urinary tract symptoms of benign prostatic hyperplasia may include the following.

- urinary frequency—urination eight or more times per day
- urinary urgency—the inability to delay urination
- difficulty starting a urine stream
- a weak or interrupted urine stream
- dribbling at the end of urination
- nocturia—frequent urination during periods of sleep
- urinary retention
- urinary incontinence—accidental loss of urine
- pain after ejaculation or during urination

The most common cause of benign prostatic hyperplasia symptoms is

- a blocked urethra

- an overworked bladder as a result of attempting to pass urine through the blockage

The severity of the blockage or discomfort is not always determined by the size of the prostate. Some men with significantly enlarged prostates have little blockage and few symptoms, whereas others with minimally enlarged prostates have more blockage and symptoms. Lower urinary tract symptoms affect less than half of all men with benign prostatic hyperplasia.

Men may not realize they have a blockage until they are unable to urinate. This disease, known as acute urinary retention, can be caused by using over-the-counter cold or allergy drugs containing decongestants such pseudoephedrine or oxymetazoline.

One of these drugs' potential negative effects is that it prevents the bladder neck from relaxing and discharging urine. Antihistamine-containing medications, such as diphenhydramine, can impair bladder muscle contraction, resulting in urine retention, difficulty urinating, and painful urination. Urinary retention can develop in men who have a partial urethra blockage as a result of alcohol use, low weather, or a protracted period of inactivity.

What are the complications of benign prostatic hyperplasia?

Benign prostatic hyperplasia consequences may include

- urinary retention (acute)
- urinary retention that is chronic or long-lasting
- urinating blood
- urinary tract infections (utis)
- bladder damage
- renal disease
- bladder stones

The majority of men with benign prostatic hyperplasia do not experience these consequences. However, when kidney impairment occurs, it can pose a major health risk.

How is benign prostatic hyperplasia diagnosed?

A healthcare practitioner determines benign prostatic hyperplasia based on the symptoms.

Personal and Family Medical History

One of the first steps a healthcare practitioner may take to assist in identifying benign prostatic hyperplasia is to obtain a personal and family medical history. A doctor may inquire about a man's health.

- what symptoms are present; when the symptoms began and how frequently they occur; whether he has a history of recurrent UTIs; and what medications, both prescription and over-the-counter, he uses.
- how much liquid he drinks on a daily basis;
- whether he uses caffeine or alcohol; and
- his general medical history, including any important illnesses or surgeries.

Physical Exam

A physical examination may aid in the diagnosis of benign prostatic hyperplasia. During a physical examination, a healthcare practitioner will most likely

- checks a patient's body, which may involve looking for urethral discharge, enlarged or tender lymph nodes in the groin, and a swollen or tender scrotum.
- taps on specific bodily parts of the patient
- does a digital rectal exam.

A digital rectal exam, or rectal exam, is a physical examination of the prostate. To conduct the exam, the doctor has the man bend over a table or lie on his side with his knees close to his chest. The doctor inserts a gloved, lubricated finger into the rectum and feels the part of the prostate adjacent to the rectum. During the rectal exam, the guy may experience minor discomfort.

A rectal exam is typically performed during an office visit by a health care professional, and men do not require anesthetic.

The exam allows the doctor to see if the prostate is swollen or sensitive, or if there are any abnormalities that necessitate further testing.

Medical Tests

Although a health care provider may send men to a urologist (a doctor who specializes in urinary disorders and the male reproductive system), the health care provider most typically diagnoses benign prostatic hyperplasia based on symptoms and a digital rectal exam.

A urologist utilizes medical testing to assist in diagnosing and treat lower urinary tract problems caused by benign prostatic hyperplasia. Medical examinations may involve.

Urinalysis

Urinalysis is the testing of a urine sample. In a health care provider's office or a commercial facility, the patient collects a urine sample in a particular container.

During an office visit, a health care professional analyses the sample or sends it to a lab for analysis. A nurse or technician performs the test by inserting a strip of chemically treated paper, known as a dipstick, into the urine. The color of the dipstick patches changes to show the presence of infection in the urine.

PSA blood test

PSA is a protein produced by prostate cells. Prostate cancer patients may have increased levels of PSA in their blood. A high PSA level, on the other hand, does not always indicate prostate cancer.

In fact, high PSA levels are frequently caused by benign prostatic hyperplasia, prostate infections, inflammation, age, and normal variations.

Much is uncertain about how to interpret a PSA blood test, the test's capacity to distinguish between cancer and benign prostatic hyperplasia, and the best course of action to take if the PSA level is high.

Urodynamic tests

Urodynamic tests are a group of techniques used to assess how well the bladder and urethra hold and discharge urine.

Urodynamic tests are performed by a health care professional at an office visit, an outpatient clinic, or a hospital. Some urodynamic tests are performed without anaesthetic, while others may require local anesthetic. The majority of urodynamic tests concentrate on the bladder's ability to hold urine and empty it steadily and completely, and may include the following:

Uroflowmetry, which assesses how quickly the bladder releases pee postvoid residual measurement, which assesses how much urine remains in the bladder after urination reduced urine flow or residual urine in the bladder, which frequently indicates urinary obstruction due to benign prostatic hyperplasia.

Cystoscopy

Cystoscopy is a procedure that employs a tube-like equipment called a cystoscope to see inside the urethra and bladder. A urologist puts the cystoscope through the hole at the tip of the penis and into the lower urinary system. A urologist does a cystoscopy at an office visit, an outpatient clinic, or a hospital.

The urologist will administer local anesthetic to the patient; but, in some circumstances, sedation and regional or general anesthesia may be required. A urologist may use cystoscopy to examine for blockages or stones in the urinary tract.

Transrectal ultrasound

Transrectal ultrasonography employs a transducer, which bounces harmless, painless sound waves off organs to produce an image of their anatomy.

To evaluate different organs, the health care provider might move the transducer to different angles. The treatment is performed in a health care provider's office, an outpatient center, or a hospital by a properly trained technician, and the images are interpreted by a radiologist—a doctor who specializes in medical imaging; the patient is not sedated. Transrectal ultrasonography is the most common method used by urologists to assess the prostate. The technician puts a transducer slightly larger than a pen into the man's rectum, adjacent to the prostate, during a transrectal ultrasonography. The ultrasound scan displays the prostate's size as well as any anomalies, such as malignancies. Transrectal ultrasonography is ineffective in detecting prostate cancer.

Biopsy

A biopsy is a process in which a small piece of prostate tissue is removed for examination under a microscope.

In an outpatient center or a hospital, the biopsy is performed by a urologist.

The urologist will administer light sedation and local anesthetic to the patient; but, in some circumstances, general anesthesia will be required. The urologist guides the biopsy needle into the prostate using imaging modalities such as ultrasound, computed tomography, or magnetic resonance imaging. In a lab, a pathologist (a specialist who specializes in studying tissues to diagnose diseases) analyzes prostate tissue. The test can determine whether or not prostate cancer is present.

Chapter 4

What is prostate cancer?

Prostate cancer occurs when abnormal cells in the prostate gland expand uncontrollably, resulting in the formation of a malignant tumor.

Prostate cancer is a type of cancer that develops in the prostate. The prostate is a small walnut-shaped gland in males that produces seminal fluid, which nourishes and transports sperm.

One of the most common types of cancer is prostate cancer. Many prostate cancers grow slowly and are restricted to the prostate gland, where they may not cause significant harm. While some types of prostate cancer develop slowly and may require little or no therapy, others are aggressive and spread quickly.

Prostate cancer that is identified early, while it is still localized to the prostate gland, has the best chance of being treated successfully.

Prostate cancer is the most commonly diagnosed cancer among men in the world.

How prostate cancer happens

Prostate cancer develops when cells in the prostate gland divide and expand uncontrolled. In males, the prostate gland is a tiny, walnut-shaped gland found underneath the bladder. It generates a fluid that feeds and transports sperm.

Prostate cancer frequently begins as neoplastic alterations in the prostate gland cells. These aberrant cells can grow into a tumor over time. Localized prostate cancer occurs when the tumor remains restricted to the prostate.

1. Genetic and Molecular Alterations

Prostate cancer typically begins with genetic and molecular changes in the prostate gland's cells. Certain genes that regulate cell growth and division can be mutated, resulting in uncontrolled cell proliferation.

2. The Influence of Androgen Hormones

Androgen hormones, such as testosterone, play an important role in the development of prostate cancer. Androgens activate prostate cancer cells, causing tumor growth. As a result, therapies that target androgen receptors are critical in illness management.

3. Age and Family Background:

Age is a major risk factor for prostate cancer. The risk of having prostate cancer increases as men age. Having a family history of prostate cancer can also increase one's risk.

4. Infections and Inflammation

Chronic inflammation and infections in the prostate may lead to prostate cancer development. According to some research, chronic inflammation may foster cancer growth.

5. Factors of Lifestyle

Certain lifestyle factors can increase one's risk of developing prostate cancer. Obesity, sedentary lifestyle, and smoking may all raise the risk of developing prostate cancer.

6. Heritable Factors

In some cases, hereditary gene mutations, such as BRCA1 and BRCA2, have been related to prostate cancer. Men who have certain genetic abnormalities are at a higher risk of getting aggressive prostate cancer.

Prostate cancer develops due to a complex interaction of genetic, hormonal, and environmental factors. While age, family history, and hereditary factors cannot be modified, a healthy lifestyle and inflammatory management may minimize the risk. Regular prostate screenings and early detection are critical for accurate diagnosis and therapy. Men can take charge of their prostate health and improve their well-being by being aware and proactive.

Although the precise origin of prostate cancer is unknown, many risk factors have been found.

One of the most important risk factors is age, with males over 65 accounting for the vast majority of cases. A close male relative with prostate cancer enhances the risks of developing the condition, as does family history and genetics.

Hormones, especially the male hormone testosterone, are thought to have a role in the development of cancer of the prostate. Both normal and malignant prostate cells proliferate in response to testosterone. As a result, men with higher testosterone levels or certain abnormalities in hormone receptors may be at greater risk. Exposure to certain chemicals, for example, has also been related to an increased risk of prostate cancer. Exposure to certain substances, such as pesticides, and air pollution are examples of environmental variables. Furthermore, food can have a role in the development of prostate cancer, with diets heavy in saturated fats and red meat being associated with an increased risk. Finally, obesity may increase the risk of prostate cancer by increasing levels of hormones such as oestrogen, which can accelerate the growth of prostate cancer cells.

Prostate cancer is a dangerous disease that should not be underestimated. However, by recognizing the disease's risk factors, it is feasible to lower the risk and improve the odds of successful treatment.

Symptoms and Signs

Symptoms are physical changes that you can notice in your body. Changes in something measured, such as your blood pressure or a lab result, are signs. Symptoms and indicators, when combined, can assist in describing a medical situation. While most prostate cancers are asymptomatic, the following symptoms and indicators of prostate cancer may occur:

- Excessive urination

- Inadequate or interrupted urine flow, as well as the need to struggle to empty the bladder

- The need to urinate repeatedly during the night

- Urine containing blood

- The emergence of new erectile dysfunction

- Urinary pain or burning, which is far less prevalent

- Sitting discomfort or pain caused by an enlarged prostate

Similar symptoms can be caused by noncancerous prostate disorders such as benign prostatic hypertrophy (BPH) or an enlarged prostate. Alternatively, the reason of a symptom or sign could be another medical disease unrelated to cancer. Urinary symptoms might also be caused by a bladder infection or other illnesses.

If cancer has gone beyond the prostate gland, the following symptoms and indicators may occur:

- Back, hip, thigh, shoulder, or other bone pain

- Swelling or fluid accumulation in the legs or feet

- Unknown cause of weight loss

- Tiredness

- Alteration in bowel habits

If you are concerned about any changes you notice, please consult your doctor. In addition to other questions, your doctor will inquire how long and how frequently you have been experiencing the symptom(s). This is done to assist in determining the cause of the condition, which is referred to as a diagnostic.

If cancer is discovered, symptom relief is an important element of cancer care and treatment. Symptom management may be referred to as "palliative care" or "supportive care." It is frequently initiated shortly after diagnosis and continues throughout treatment. Make an appointment with your healthcare provider to discuss your symptoms, particularly any new or changing symptoms.

Chapter 5

What is Advanced Prostate Cancer?

When prostate cancer spreads beyond the prostate or returns after treatment, it is referred to as advanced prostate cancer.

Advanced prostate cancer, also known as metastatic prostate cancer, is a stage of prostate cancer in which cancer cells have moved outside of the prostate gland to other areas of the body. Prostate cancer is one of the most frequent malignancies in men, and when it progresses, it can provide substantial treatment and management issues.

There are various forms of advanced prostate cancer;

Biochemical Recurrence:

With biochemical recurrence, the prostate-specific antigen (PSA) level has increased following treatment(s) with surgery or radiation, but no other signs of cancer have been found.

Castration-Resistant Prostate Cancer (CRPC):

Castration-resistant prostate cancer (CRPC) is an advanced stage of prostate cancer. CRPC indicates that the prostate cancer is developing or spreading despite decreased testosterone levels caused by hormone therapy. Hormone therapy, also known as testosterone depletion therapy or androgen deprivation treatment (ADT), can help reduce your natural testosterone level. Most men with prostate cancer are given either medicine or surgery to diminish the testosterone "fuel" that causes cancer to develop. This fuel consists of male hormones or androgens (such as testosterone). Hormone therapy typically suppresses prostate cancer growth, at least temporarily. If cancer cells learn to "outsmart" hormone therapy, they can thrive even in the absence of testosterone. If this occurs, the prostate cancer is classified as CRPC.

Non-Metastatic Castration-Resistant Prostate Cancer (nmCRPC):

Prostate cancer that is only detected in the prostate and no longer responds to hormone treatment.

This is indicated by an increase in PSA levels while testosterone levels remain low. Imaging tests do not reveal evidence of cancer metastasis.

Metastatic Prostate Cancer (MPC):

Metastasis is a key and complex process in cancer that occurs when cancer cells move from the initial tumor site to other parts of the body, establishing secondary tumors in distant organs or tissues and traveling through the bloodstream or lymphatic system. The bones, lymph nodes, liver, and lungs are common sites of metastasis.

You may be diagnosed with metastatic prostate cancer when you are first diagnosed, after your initial therapy, or even many years afterward. It is unusual to be diagnosed with metastatic prostate cancer for the first time, but it does occur.

Metastatic Hormone-Sensitive Prostate Cancer (mHSPC):

Metastatic hormone-sensitive prostate cancer (mHSPC) occurs when cancer has gone beyond the prostate throughout the body and is responsive to hormone therapy, or when the patient is yet to undergo hormone therapy. This means that levels of male sex hormones, particularly androgens like testosterone, can be decreased to prevent the progression of cancer. If left unchecked, these male sex hormones "feed" prostate cancer cells, allowing them to develop. Hormone therapy, such as ADT, may be used to lower these hormone levels.

Metastatic Castration-Resistant Prostate Cancer (mCRPC):

Metastatic castration-resistant prostate cancer occurs when cancer has migrated beyond the prostate and continues to develop and spread even after testosterone-lowering treatments have been utilized. PSA values continue to rise, and metastatic areas are present/growing. Despite medicinal or surgical castration, this is disease progression.

Mechanism: Metastasis is the process by which cancer cells spread to a new location:

- **Invasion**: Cancer cells first invade adjacent tissues by breaching the tissue boundaries.

- **Intravasation**: Some cancer cells penetrate neighboring blood vessels (intravasate) or lymphatic vessels (lymphovasate), allowing them to migrate through the circulation or lymphatic system.

- **Circulation**: Cancer cells in the bloodstream or lymphatic system travel to distant parts of the body such as the bones, liver, lungs, brain, and other organs.

- **Arrest and Extravasation**: Cancer cells become caught in the small blood arteries of distant organs, where they can leave (extravasate) and form secondary tumors.

- **Formation of Secondary Tumors**: Cancer cells can replicate and grow after leaving the bloodstream, producing secondary tumors in fresh tissue.

Factors Affecting Metastasis: Several factors influence cancer cells' capacity to metastasize, including the type of cancer, the aggressiveness of the tumor, the presence of specific genetic abnormalities, and the overall health of the patient's immune system.

prostate cancer is graded using the Gleason score, which assesses the aggressiveness of cancer cells based on their microscopic appearance. The TNM staging approach, on the other hand, categorizes prostate cancer based on the amount of the tumor inside the prostate, the involvement of lymph nodes, and the evidence of distant metastases. These grading and staging systems work together to help healthcare professionals select the best treatment option for men with prostate cancer. Early identification, as well as precise grading and staging, are critical for making informed treatment decisions and predicting prognosis.

Chapter 6

Prostate Grading and Staging

The extent and aggressiveness of the cancer cells are often used to classify and grade prostate cancer. The stages are determined by the amount and rate at which the cancer cells grow. The Gleason score and the T (tumor), N (node), and M (metastasis) staging system are the two main approaches used to classify prostate cancer. Let's take a closer look at these:

1. Gleason Score

The Gleason score is a classification system that evaluates the microscopic appearance of prostate cancer cells in a biopsy sample. It is commonly used to assess the aggressiveness of prostate cancer. The Gleason score is determined by the pattern of cancer cell proliferation and is commonly expressed as a sum of two values ranging from 2 to 10.

- Low-grade cancers with Gleason scores ranging from 2 to 6. These tumors are well-differentiated, which means the cancer cells resemble normal prostate cells and are less aggressive.
- Intermediate-grade cancers have a Gleason score of 7. These tumors show a moderate level of differentiation and can be classified as 3+4 (less aggressive) or 4+3 (more aggressive).
- Gleason scores of 8 to 10 for high-grade cancers. These tumors are less differentiated, with cells that bear little resemblance to normal prostate cells and are often more aggressive.

A higher Gleason score suggests that the cancer is more likely to develop and spread quickly.

2. TNM Staging System

The TNM staging method describes the degree and spread of prostate cancer based on three important factors:

T (Tumor): The size and extent of the main tumor within the prostate gland are indicated by this letter. T1 (early and palpable), T2 (limited to the prostate), T3 (extending beyond the prostate), and T4 (invading neighboring structures) are the most common classifications.

N (Nodes): Indicates whether the malignancy has spread to surrounding lymph nodes. It is classed as N0 (no lymph node involvement) or N1 (regional lymph node involvement).

M (Metastasis): Indicates whether the cancer has migrated to other organs such as the bones, liver, or lungs. It is classed as M0 (no distant metastasis) or M1 (existing distant metastasis).

When the T, N, and M categories are combined, an overall stage classification (e.g., Stage I, II, III, or IV) is produced, which aids in determining the degree of the disease and guiding treatment recommendations.

- Stages I and II: The tumor has not spread beyond the prostate.
- Locally Advanced | Stage III: Cancer has spread outside the prostate but only to adjacent tissues.
- Advanced | Stage IV: Cancer has spread outside the prostate to other organs such as the lymph nodes, bones, liver, or lungs.

Prostate Cancer Stage Groupings

Prostate cancer is classified as follows:

T: The health care provider cannot feel the tumor.

T1: Cancer found in less than 5% of excised tissue and of low grade (Gleason less than 6).

T2: Cancer that has spread to more than 5% of the excised tissue or is of a higher grade (Gleason score greater than 6).

T3: Cancer discovered via needle biopsy as a result of a high PSA.

T4: The doctor can feel the tumor with a DRE, but it is only in the prostate.

T5: Cancer identified in one half or less of one side (left or right) of the prostate.

T6: Cancer diagnosed on more than half of one side (left or right) of the prostate.

T7: Cancer present on both sides of the prostate.

T8: Cancer has gone beyond the prostate and may have affected the seminal vesicles.

T9: Cancer spreads beyond the prostate but does not reach the seminal vesicles.

T10: Cancer has expanded to the seminal vesicles, according to

T11: Cancer has spread to neighboring organs.

N0: There is no evidence of cancer spreading to the lymph nodes in the prostate area (becomes N1 if cancer has spread to lymph nodes).

M0: No evidence of tumor metastasis (M1 if cancer has spread to other areas of the body).

What are the stages of prostate cancer and their implications?

Prostate cancer is a form of cancer that most commonly occurs in the prostate gland, a small walnut-shaped organ in the male reproductive system. The stages of prostate cancer show the amount and spread of the disease, which helps decide effective treatment options and estimate the patient's prognosis.

Stage I: At this early stage, the cancer is restricted to a small area of the prostate gland and is usually slow-growing. The implications of stage I prostate cancer are generally good, as it is highly treated with a high probability of cure.

Stage II: The cancer has spread beyond the boundaries of the prostate but remains contained within the gland. The consequences are determined by criteria such as the tumor's size and the Gleason score (a measure of the cancer's aggressiveness). There are therapy alternatives available, and the chances of effective treatment and survival are high.

Stage III: The cancer has gone beyond the prostate gland and may have infiltrated surrounding tissues such as the seminal vesicles. The consequences of stage III prostate cancer show that the cancer is more likely to move to lymph nodes or other distant organs. Surgery, radiation therapy, hormone therapy, or a combination of these may be used as treatment options.

Stage IV: The cancer has progressed to distant organs such as the bones, liver, or lungs at this point. At this stage, the consequences are more severe, and the therapeutic focus switches to illness management rather than curative aim. Treatment options may include radiation therapy, chemotherapy, hormone therapy, or immunotherapy, depending on the individual instance.

Chapter 7

Diagnosis and Biopsy

Prostate cancer is normally diagnosed using a combination of medical history, physical examination, and several diagnostic tests. Several tests are performed to determine whether cancer has spread to another place of the body from where it began. Metastasis refers to the spread of cancer. Tests and analyses may also be performed to determine which therapies are most likely to be effective.

How prostate cancer is diagnosed

There are numerous tests available to diagnose prostate cancer. Not all of the tests described here are typically utilized for every individual. When selecting a diagnostic test, your doctor may take the following considerations into account:

- The sort of cancer that is suspected

- Describe your indications and symptoms.

- Your age and general well-being

• The outcomes of previous medical tests

Early tests

If prostate cancer is suspected, a physical exam and the following tests may be done to determine whether more diagnostic testing are required:

Prostate-Specific Antigen (PSA) Test

PSA is a protein produced by prostate tissue that is present in higher concentrations in the blood. When there is aberrant activity in the prostate, such as prostate cancer, benign prostatic hypertrophy (BPH), or inflammation of the prostate, levels might rise. Doctors can use PSA value characteristics such as absolute level, change over time (also known as "PSA velocity"), and level in relation to prostate size to determine whether a biopsy is necessary.

A blood test detects PSA, a protein generated by the prostate gland. PSA values that are elevated can be indicative of prostate issues, but they do not definitively identify prostate cancer. Other disorders, such as benign prostatic hyperplasia (BPH), also induce increased PSA values.

Free PSA test

The "free" PSA test is a variation of the PSA test that allows the clinician to measure a specific component. PSA is present free in the bloodstream and is not linked to proteins. A conventional PSA test examines total PSA, which includes both PSA that is and is not coupled to proteins. The free PSA test calculates the free PSA/total PSA ratio. Knowing this ratio or percentage can sometimes assist in determining whether an increased PSA result is more likely to be connected with a malignant condition such as prostate cancer.

Digital Rectal Examination (DRE)

The doctor uses a greased, gloved finger to feel the prostate gland during a DRE.

This can aid in the detection of any anomalies or suspicious lumps. Because it is not extremely exact and not every doctor is trained in it, DRE does not frequently detect early prostate cancer.

Medical History and Symptoms Assessment

Your doctor will begin by getting a thorough medical history, including any family history of prostate cancer or other pertinent cancers.

You'll be asked about any symptoms you're having, such as urinary issues (frequent urination, difficulty starting or stopping urination, weak urine flow), blood in the urine or sperm, pain in the lower back, pelvic, or hips, or erectile dysfunction.

Imaging Tests

Imaging studies may be conducted if prostate cancer is suspected or confirmed to identify the extent of the cancer and whether it has spread to other places of the body. Typical imaging tests include:

Transrectal Ultrasound (TRUS)

Sound waves are used to make images of the prostate gland in this process.
A doctor inserts a probe into the rectum and uses sound waves that bounce off the prostate to create an image of the prostate.

MRI (Magnetic Resonance Imaging)

MRI scans produce very detailed images of the prostate and its surrounding tissues.

An MRI scan produces detailed images of the body by using magnetic fields rather than x-rays. An MRI can be used to determine the size of the tumor, and the scan can be focused on the prostate or the entire body. To provide a clearer image, a special dye called contrast medium is injected into a patient's vein before to the scan.

CT (Computed Tomography) Scan

CT scans can assist in detecting metastases in lymph nodes and distant organs.

A CT scan uses X-rays captured from various angles to create images of the inside of the body. A computer combines these images to create a detailed, three-dimensional image of any anomalies or malignancies. A CT scan can be performed to determine the size of the tumor. To improve image detail, a specific dye known as a contrast medium is sometimes administered prior to the scan. This dye can be injected into a patient's vein or administered orally as a tablet or drink.

Prostate biopsy

Prostate gland biopsy; transrectal prostate biopsy; fine needle prostate biopsy; core prostate biopsy; Prostate biopsy with a specific goal in mind; Prostate biopsy - transrectal ultrasonography (TRUS); stereotactic transperineal prostate biopsy (STPB).

What exactly is a prostate biopsy?

A prostate biopsy is the removal of small samples of tissue from the prostate gland with a fine needle in order to look for evidence of prostate cancer.

How the Test Is Conducted

A prostate biopsy can be performed in three ways.

Transrectal prostate biopsy entails taking a biopsy through the rectum. This is the most widely used approach.

You will be asked to lie down on your side, knees bent.

A finger-sized ultrasound probe will be inserted into your rectum by your doctor. You might feel some discomfort or pressure.

The provider can see images of the prostate thanks to the ultrasound. Using these photos, the practitioner will inject a numbing drug around the prostate.

The provider will then inject the biopsy needle into the prostate to take a sample, using ultrasonography to guide the needle. A short stinging sensation may result.

A total of 10 to 18 samples will be collected. They will be examined in the laboratory.

The complete procedure should take no more than 10 minutes.

Other prostate biopsy procedures are utilized, albeit seldom. These are some examples:

Transurethral - through the urethra.

You will be given medication to make you asleep so that you do not experience any discomfort.

A flexible tube with a camera on the end (cystoscope) is introduced via the urethral opening at the penis's tip.
The scope is used to collect tissue samples from the prostate.

Perineal refers to the skin between the anus and the scrotum.

You will be given medication to make you asleep so that you do not experience any discomfort.
A needle is introduced into the perineum to collect prostate tissue.

Why Biopsy is Performed

A biopsy is carried out for a variety of medical reasons, the most common of which is to diagnose or confirm the presence of diseases or ailments within the body. A small sample of tissue or cells is removed from a specified area of the body for examination under a microscope.

If your doctor suggests a prostate biopsy, it is because:

A blood test reveals that you have higher-than-normal prostate specific antigen (PSA) levels.

During a digital rectal exam, your provider discovers a lump or irregularity in your prostate.

Diagnosis of Cancer

Cancer is routinely diagnosed through biopsies. Doctors can identify whether cancer is present, the type of cancer, the stage of the disease, and the aggressiveness of the cancer by studying the tissue or cells from a suspicious growth or lump. Breast biopsies, prostate biopsies, and skin biopsies are among examples.

Evaluation of Tissue Abnormalities

When there are aberrant tissue changes or lesions that are not explained by conventional diagnostic testing, a biopsy can help pinpoint the cause of the anomaly. This is common in skin disorders, mouth lesions, and gastrointestinal problems.

Assessment of Infections

Biopsies can detect the presence of infectious pathogens within tissues, such as bacteria, viruses, or fungi. This is critical for detecting diseases such as tuberculosis, fungal infections, and viral hepatitis.

Characterization of Inflammatory Conditions

Biopsies can be used to identify and evaluate inflammatory diseases such as autoimmune disorders, which can assist in determining the extent of tissue damage and guide therapy options.

Evaluation of Organ Function

Biopsies of organs such as the liver, kidney, or heart may be performed to evaluate their function and detect abnormalities or disorders such as hepatitis, cirrhosis, or cardiomyopathy.

Identification of Genetic or Molecular Abnormalities: Genetic or molecular testing on biopsy samples may be undertaken in some situations to identify specific genetic abnormalities, markers, or biomarkers linked with specific diseases or disorders. This data can be used to inform treatment decisions and personalized medical techniques.

Monitoring Treatment Progress

Biopsies may be repeated during or after therapy to evaluate the efficacy of treatments and to identify whether the disease has reacted or worsened.

Surgical Planning Advice

Biopsies can assist surgeons in treatment planning by providing information about the kind and size of a lesion or tumor, allowing them to determine the optimal surgical strategy.

Research and Clinical Trials

Biopsies are essential in medical research and clinical trials aimed at better-understanding diseases, generating new medicines, and assessing treatment outcomes.

How the Test will Feel

During the procedure you may feel:
- Mild discomfort as the probe is placed
- A brief sting when the biopsy needle is used to collect a sample

- Following the procedure, you may experience:
- Rectal soreness
- Small amounts of blood in your feces, urine, or sperm, which might linger for days to weeks
- Light rectum bleeding
- Your clinician may recommend antibiotics to take for several days following the biopsy to avoid infection. Make careful to take the entire dose as directed.

How to Prepare for the Test

Your provider will explain the risks and advantages of the biopsy to you. You may be required to sign a consent form.

- Your provider may advise you to stop taking any of the following medications several days before the biopsy:

- Warfarin (Coumadin, Jantoven), clopidogrel (Plavix), apixaban (Eliquis), dabigatran (Pradaxa), edoxaban (Savaysa), rivaroxaban (Xarelto), or aspirin-based nonsteroidal anti-inflammatory medications (NSAIDs) such as aspirin and ibuprofen
- Supplements made from herbs
- Vitamins
- Continue to take any prescription medications unless your provider instructs you otherwise.

- Your provider may request that you:
- The day before the biopsy, eat only light meals.
- Before the treatment, perform an enema at home to cleanse your rectum.
- Antibiotics should be taken the day before, the day of, and the day after your biopsy.

Danger of Prostate Biopsy

A prostate biopsy is generally safe, however there are some dangers involved, such as infection or sepsis (severe blood infection). Having difficulty passing urine, an adverse reaction to medications, and bleeding or bruising at the biopsy site are all possibilities.

Do You Really Need a Prostate Exam?

A prostate exam, which commonly involves a DRE and a Prostate-Specific Antigen (PSA) blood test, is not required for all men. Whether or not to have a prostate exam is a personal decision based on personal variables and preferences.

Many men are hesitant to undergo prostate cancer screening, particularly a rectal exam. True, this exam is slightly intrusive; nevertheless, it is brief and typically painless. While the PSA blood test can detect many prostate tumors, there are those that can only be discovered by a rectal exam. Screening enables for the earlier discovery of the disease, making treatment much easier.

One difficulty with prostate cancer is that the early stages sometimes present with no symptoms, which is why annual screening checks are critical. Once prostate cancer has metastasized and spread to other parts of the body, it is usually incurable.

Prostate cancer screening should begin at the age of 55 for men who are at average risk. Screening is generally not advised in men over the age of 75 because the possible benefits exceed the hazards in this cohort. Men at high risk should begin screenings at the age of 45. Patients with a strong family history are at higher risk of more aggressive illness.

Where does prostate cancer spread?

If prostate cancer is not detected and treated early, it can spread (metastasize) to other regions of the body.

Prostate cancer metastasis occurs when cells in the prostate break away from the tumor. Cancer cells can spread to other parts of the body via the lymphatic system or circulation. The following are the most prevalent areas where prostate cancer can spread:

1. Lymph Nodes: Prostate cancer can spread to neighboring lymph nodes in the pelvic area. Enlarged or atypical lymph nodes seen during imaging or surgery may suggest cancer spread.

2. Bones: Bone metastases are a common site for prostate cancer spread. It can affect bones such as the spine, hips, pelvis, and ribs. Bone metastases can cause pain, fractures, and other consequences.

3. Other Organs: Although prostate cancer is uncommon, it can spread to other organs such as the liver, lungs, and, in rare cases, the brain. Metastasis in various organs can cause symptoms unique to the organ in question.

Chapter 8

Treatment and Side Effects

Prostate cancer is the most frequent cancer among men. The best treatment depends on the stage of the cancer, the patient's overall health, and personal preferences.

The goal of advanced prostate cancer treatment is to reduce or control tumor development as well as to alleviate symptoms. There are numerous therapy options available for advanced prostate cancer. Which treatment to use and when will be determined by discussions with your doctor. Before deciding on a treatment plan, consult with your doctor about how to address adverse effects.

What is Hormone Therapy?

Hormone therapy is a treatment that reduces a man's testosterone levels. This therapy is also known as ADT. Because testosterone, a crucial male sex hormone, is the primary fuel for prostate cancer cells, lowering its levels may halt their growth.

Hormone therapy may help decrease prostate cancer growth in men whose cancer has metastasized (spread) away from the prostate or reappeared after prior therapies. Some treatments may be used to decrease or control a non-spreading local tumor. Hormone therapy for prostate cancer treatment comes in a variety of forms, including drugs and surgery.

Hormone Therapy with Surgery

The removal of the testicles for hormone therapy is known as orchiectomy or castration. When the testicles are removed, the body is unable to produce the hormones that feed prostate cancer. In the United States, it is rarely used as a therapy option. Men who select this therapy want a one-time surgical procedure. They must be willing to have their testicles permanently removed and be in good enough health to undergo surgery.

There are numerous advantages to having an orchiectomy to treat advanced prostate cancer. It is not costly. It is straightforward and has low dangers.

It only needs to be done once. It is immediately effective. Testosterone levels plummet precipitously.

Side Effects

Infection and bleeding are two possible side effects for your body. Because removing the testicles causes the body to stop producing testosterone, there is a risk of the hormone therapy adverse effects described below. Other adverse effects of this operation may be related to body image because of the appearance of the genital area following surgery. To help the scrotum resemble the same as before surgery, some men prefer to have artificial testicles or saline implants. Some men choose a procedure known as subcapsular orchiectomy. This removes the glands inside the testicles but leaves the testicles themselves intact, resulting in a normal-looking scrotum.

Hormone Therapy with Medications

Hormone therapy is offered in several forms, including injections and pills that can be taken orally. Some of these treatments inhibit the body's production of a luteinizing hormone-releasing hormone (LHRH, also known as gonadotrophin-releasing hormone or GnRH).

LHRH stimulates the body's production of testosterone. Other medications, such as inhibiting hormone receptors, prevent testosterone from affecting prostate cells. A blood test is sometimes performed after the first shot. This test is used to determine testosterone levels. During therapy, you may also be subjected to tests to assess your bone density.

There is no need for surgery with LHRH therapy. Men who are unable or unwilling to have their testicles removed may be candidates for this procedure.

Your doctor may prescribe one of several types of medicinal hormone therapy to reduce your body's testosterone production. You are at a "castration level" when your testosterone levels are extremely low.

Prostate cancer cells' growth and proliferation may slow as testosterone levels fall.

Types of Medications

Agonists (analogs)

LHRH/GnRH agonists are medications that reduce testosterone levels. They could be used to treat cancer that has returned, whether or not it has spread.

Agonists stimulate the body to release a burst of testosterone (known as a "flare") when initially administered. Agonists last longer than natural LHRH. Following the initial flare, the medicine tricks your brain into thinking it doesn't need to create LHRH/GnRH because it already has plenty. As a result, the testicles are not stimulated to make testosterone.

LHRH or GnRH agonists are administered as injections or as tiny pellets injected beneath the skin. They could be administered once every one, three, or six months, depending on the medicine.

Antagonists

These medications also reduce testosterone levels. Rather than overwhelming the pituitary gland with LHRH, they prevent it from attaching to receptors. There is no testosterone flare when using an LHRH/GnRH antagonist since the body does not get the signal to create testosterone.

Antibodies can be taken orally or injected (shot) beneath the skin, buttocks, or abdomen. The shot is administered in the doctor's office. You will most likely be asked to stay in the office for a bit after the shot to verify there is no allergic response.

A blood test is performed after the first shot to ensure that testosterone levels have decreased. You may also be subjected to bone density tests.

Anti-androgen drugs

Antiandrogen medications are taken orally as pills. This therapy is partially dependent on where the cancer has progressed and its consequences.

This medication reduces testosterone levels by blocking androgen receptors in prostate cancer cells. Normally, testosterone binds to these receptors to promote the growth of prostate cancer cells. When the receptors are inhibited, testosterone is unable to "feed" the prostate. Anti-androgen medication used a few weeks before or after LHRH therapy may minimize "flare-ups." Antiandrogens may also be utilized after surgery or castration if hormone therapy is no longer effective.

CAB (combination androgen-reduction therapy with anti-androgens)

This method combines castration (either surgically or with the medications mentioned above) and antiandrogen drugs. The medication decreases testosterone synthesis and can help prevent it from attaching to cancer cells.

Surgery or oral medications may be used to reduce the amount of testosterone produced by your testicles. The adrenal glands produce the remaining testosterone. Antiandrogen therapy inhibits the production of testosterone by the adrenal glands.

Androgen synthesis inhibitors

These medications work to prevent other regions of your body (as well as cancer) from producing more testosterone and its metabolites. Men with metastatic hormone-sensitive prostate cancer (mHSPC) or metastatic castration-resistant prostate cancer (mCRPC) who have just been diagnosed may be ideal candidates for this therapy.

Androgen production inhibitors are pills that can be taken orally. This medication prevents your body from producing the enzyme required to produce androgens in your adrenal glands, testicles, and prostate tissue, resulting in lower amounts of testosterone and other androgens. Because of the way it works, it must be used with an oral steroid.

Hormone Therapy Side Effects

Unfortunately, hormone therapy does not cure cancer and may not last forever. Despite the modest hormone level, the tumour may grow over time. Other therapies are required to control the malignancy.

Hormone therapy have numerous potential adverse effects. Find out what they are. Intermittent (rather than continuous) hormone therapy may potentially be an option for treatment. Consult your doctor before beginning any sort of hormone therapy.

Possible hormone therapy side effects include:

- Most guys have a lower libido (sexual desire).
- Erectile dysfunction, or the inability to obtain or maintain a strong enough erection for sex;
- Erectile dysfunction, or the inability to achieve or maintain a strong enough erection for sex;
- Hot flashes or a quick spread of heat to the face, neck, and upper torso, as well as excessive sweating
- A 10 to 15-pound weight gain. Dieting, eating fewer processed foods, and exercising may help you lose weight.
- Mood swings
- Depression, including feelings of hopelessness, loss of interest in enjoyable activities, inability to concentrate, or changes in appetite and sleeping
- Fatigue (feeling tired) that does not go away with rest or sleep
- Anemia (low red blood cell count) caused by less oxygen reaching tissues and organs, causing tiredness or weaknessLoss of muscle mass causing weakness or low strength

- Weak bones (loss of bone mineral density) or bones becoming thinner, fragile, and more easily broken
- High cholesterol, particularly LDL ("bad") cholesterol
- Breast nipple soreness or increased breast tissue growth
- Increased risk of diabetes

There are numerous advantages and disadvantages to each type of hormone therapy, so consult with your doctor to determine what is best for you.

What is Chemotherapy?

Chemotherapy medications can slow cancer growth. These medications may alleviate symptoms and lengthen life. Alternatively, they may alleviate pain and symptoms by reducing tumors.

Chemotherapy can help men whose cancer has spread to other areas of their bodies.

The majority of chemotherapy medications are administered through a vein (intravenous, IV). Chemotherapy medicines circulate throughout the body. They kill both cancer cells and non-cancer cells that are rapidly developing. Chemotherapy is not always the primary treatment for prostate cancer. However, it may be an option for men whose cancer has spread. Chemotherapy may be administered prior to the onset of pain in order to avoid pain as the cancer spreads to bones and other locations.

Hair loss, exhaustion, nausea, and vomiting are all possible side effects. Changes in your perception of taste and touch are possible. You may be more susceptible to infections. Neuropathy (tingling or numbness in the hands and feet) is possible. Because of the negative effects of chemotherapy, the decision to use these medications may be influenced by:

- Your health and your ability to tolerate the medicine
- What other treatments have you tried?

- If immediate pain relief requires radiation,
- What additional treatments and clinical trials are there?
- Your treatment objectives
- If you undergo chemotherapy, your medical team may constantly monitor you to manage side effects.

There are medications available to alleviate symptoms such as nausea. Most adverse effects disappear once chemotherapy is completed.

What is Immunotherapy?

Immunotherapy combats cancer by utilizing the body's immune system. It could be an option for males with mCRPC who have no or only mild symptoms.

If the cancer returns and spreads, your doctor may recommend a cancer vaccination to increase your immune system's ability to attack cancer cells. Immunotherapy may be administered to mCRPC patients prior to or concurrently with treatment.

Side Effects

Fever, chills, weakness, headache, nausea, vomiting, and diarrhea are common in the first 24 hours after treatment. Patients may also experience low blood pressure and skin rashes.

What is Bone-targeted Therapy?

Men with prostate cancer that has gone to the bones may benefit from bone-targeted therapy because they may experience "skeletal-related events" (SREs). Fractures, discomfort, and other issues are examples of SREs.

If you have advanced prostate cancer or are on hormone therapy, your doctor may recommend calcium, vitamin D, or other bone-building medications. These medications may help stop the cancer, reduce SREs, and avoid pain and weakness caused by cancer in your bones.

Radiopharmaceuticals are radioactive medications. They can be used to alleviate bone discomfort caused by metastatic cancer. Some of these medications may also be utilized in males whose mCRPC has spread to their bones. When ADT is not working, they may be offered. Radiopharmaceuticals emit modest amounts of radiation that target the areas of the body where cancer cells are proliferating.

SRE-lowering medications may aid in bone turnover. Low calcium levels, poor kidney function, and, in rare cases, jawbone disintegration are also possible side effects.

Calcium and vitamin D are also utilized to keep your bones healthy. They are frequently suggested for men undergoing hormone therapy for prostate cancer.

What is Radiation Therapy?

Prostate cancer frequently spreads to the bones. Radiation therapy can help relieve pain and prevent fractures caused by cancer spreading to the bone.

Radiation treatments come in a variety of forms. Radiation might be administered once or over multiple sessions. Treatment is similar to getting an x-ray. Tumors are killed with high-energy beams. Some radiation treatments are designed to preserve neighboring healthy tissue. Computers and software enable more precise planning and targeting of radiation dosages. They direct the radiation precisely where it is required.

Chapter 9

Taking Care of Your Prostate

Taking care of your prostate is a vital part of overall health, especially as you become older. While there is no sure method to prevent prostate problems, you can take proactive steps to maintain prostate health and lower your risk of certain disorders.

Dietary Choices

Are you of the age where you've started to think about your prostate health?

It's no secret that taking care of your body becomes increasingly important as you get older. And, let's be honest, a healthy prostate equals less stress and a happier existence.

The good news is that by making simple dietary changes and choosing natural supplements, you may support the health of your prostate and live life to the fullest.

1.Tomatoes

Begin your adventure by harnessing the power of tomatoes.

Tomatoes, which are high in lycopene, a potent antioxidant, have been associated with a lower incidence of prostate problems. To gain their advantages, consume them in a variety of forms, including fresh, cooked, or in sauces. Lycopene has been discovered to be anti-inflammatory, which may reduce the incidence of prostate cancer considerably.

2. Cruciferous Vegetables

Remember to incorporate cruciferous vegetables into your diet. Broccoli, cauliflower, kale, and Brussels sprouts are high in nutrients including sulforaphane, which may help keep your prostate healthy. These vegetables include chemicals such as sulforaphane, which may have anti-cancer potential.

3. Berries

Berries may add a burst of flavor and health benefits to your meals.

Blueberries, strawberries, raspberries, and blackberries are high in antioxidants, which can help protect your prostate cells from damage.

4. Healthy Fats

Choose healthy fats from fatty fish (salmon, mackerel, and trout), avocados, almonds, and olive oil. These fats contain vital omega-3 fatty acids, which are anti-inflammatory and may benefit prostate health.

5. Green Tea with Hibiscus Tea

You might wish to replace your regular beverage with a soothing cup of green tea.

Green tea includes polyphenols; it has more polyphenols than any other plant since the fermentation and oxidation process removes certain antioxidants from black and oolong tea; this potent antioxidant lowers the risk of prostate cancer.

Drink at least one cup per day, but 3-4 cups per day will provide the greatest benefit.

6. Cut back on added sugars and processed foods

Reduce your consumption of sugary drinks, sweets, and highly processed foods.

Avoid sugary liquids such as sodas and many fruit juices. Sweets are only eaten on rare occasions.

7. Foods High in Fiber

Include fiber-rich foods like whole grains (brown rice, whole wheat, oats), legumes (beans, lentils), and nuts in your meals. Fiber promotes intestinal health and can aid with weight management.

8. Proteins derived from plants

Consider introducing plant-based protein sources into your diet, such as tofu, tempeh, beans, and lentils.

Legumes, particularly isoflavone-rich whole soy products such as tofu, soy milk, edamame, and tempeh, as well as other Beans, Peas, and Lentils, are high in isoflavones.

9. Limit Red and Processed Meats

Reduce your intake of red meat (beef, pork, lamb) and processed meats (sausages, hot dogs, and bacon). Consumption of these meats in excess has been linked to an elevated risk of prostate cancer.

10. Hydration

Drink plenty of water to stay hydrated. Proper hydration benefits overall health and can aid in the maintenance of urinary function. It is recommended that you drink at least eight cups of water per day. So don't try to drink less in order to minimize your pee output.

11. Moderate Alcohol Intake

Moderate alcohol intake refers to consuming alcohol in a way that does not have an adverse effect on one's health.

If you do drink, do so in moderation. Excessive alcohol consumption is linked to an increased risk of a variety of health concerns, including prostate problems.

12. Pumpkin Seeds

When it comes to prostate health, these tiny seeds carry a big punch.

Pumpkin seeds are high in zinc, a mineral required for optimal prostate gland function. Snack on them or toss them into salads.

Pumpkin seeds are one of the healthiest snacks since they are high in key nutrients and minerals needed for the body's regular optimum functioning.

Protein is abundant in pumpkin seeds. It has a large amount of unsaturated fats, omega 6 and omega 3 fatty acids, which aid in the prevention of heart disease, high blood sugar levels, and cholesterol management. It also contains fiber, which aids digestion and provides a feeling of fullness. It is a good source of calcium for bones, iron for blood, Vitamin B12 for red blood cell development, and beta-carotene, which our bodies convert to Vitamin A. It also contains magnesium, which the body requires for protein synthesis, potassium for the proper functioning of important organs and muscles, zinc for immunity, and Vitamin K, which aids in blood clotting and prevents blood loss due to excessive bleeding.

Stay Active

Maintaining a healthy diet is only one piece of the problem. An active lifestyle is also beneficial to your prostate and general health.

It is important to understand that exercise cannot "remove" prostate problems on its own.

Regular exercise, on the other hand, can be useful for controlling prostate health and lowering the chance of acquiring certain prostate diseases.

Regular exercise relieves tension and reduces stress. It maintains appropriate hormone levels and boosts immunological function.

Even 30 minutes of moderate movement per day, such as a brisk walk or jog, might be quite beneficial. Many studies indicate that you exercise 5 days per week at a moderate intensity for at least 30 minutes.

Exercise aids in achieving and maintaining a healthy weight, which has been related to a lower risk of various prostate health conditions, including prostate cancer raises the chance of aggressive prostate cancer as well as the likelihood of dying from prostate cancer.

Some workouts that can be especially beneficial to prostate health include:

1. Kegel exercises

These exercises involve contracting and relaxing the pelvic floor muscles. Kegel exercises can help with bladder control and reduce the risk of incontinence and other urinary diseases.

2. Aerobic exercise

Walking, running, swimming, or cycling can improve cardiovascular health, which can benefit prostate health.

3. Resistance training

Lifting weights or utilizing resistance bands can help you gain muscle strength and enhance your overall physical fitness.

It is critical to check with a healthcare practitioner before beginning any new fitness regimen, especially if you have an existing prostate disease. They can make tailored recommendations based on your specific needs and medical history.

Losing weight is one of the most significant natural steps toward better prostate health, whether your concerns are cancer, BPH, or prostatitis.

Read and compare food labels to find low-sodium options. Reduce your intake of canned, processed, and frozen foods.

These bad diets might raise your chances of getting an enlarged prostate and aggravate current prostate problems.

Quit addictions

Smoking both cigarettes and marijuana raises the risk of prostate cancer and other prostate-related disorders by changing hormone levels and exposing one to carcinogens. It can also increase the number of urinary tract infections.

Similarly, alcohol and caffeine can produce unfavorable inflammation in the body. To have a healthy prostate, you should avoid or reduce your addictions.

Stress Reduction

Long-term stress can weaken the immune system, disrupt hormonal balance, and make you more prone to disease.

Prostate disease can also increase your worry and anxiety, which can worsen the situation because stress interferes with the immune system's ability to fight the illness. As a result, stress management is critical.

Screening

The initial prostate test, usually performed around the age of 40, helps to establish a baseline "normal" number that is unique to the individual. raises the chance of aggressive prostate cancer as well as the likelihood of dying from prostate cancer, according to research.

Prostate cancer screening recommendations vary depending on risk group, according to the Centers for Disease Control and Prevention. African Americans, persons of Scandinavian heritage, and anyone with two or more family members diagnosed with prostate cancer should consider getting examined for prostate cancer starting at the age of 40. Men who are at normal risk are urged to begin tests at the age of 55.

Screenings may include a digital rectal exam and a blood test for prostate-specific antigen (PSA).

Quercetin Prostate

Quercetin is a flavonoid, a natural plant chemical present in a variety of fruits, vegetables, and other plant-based meals. It has gotten a lot of interest because of its possible health advantages, especially its involvement in prostate health. Here is an overview of quercetin and its potential impact on prostate health.

Here's a primer on quercetin and how it might affect prostate health:

1. Antioxidant Properties: Quercetin is a powerful antioxidant, which means it helps the body neutralize damaging free radicals. Free radical-induced oxidative stress can contribute to a variety of health conditions, including prostate problems.

2. Anti-Inflammatory qualities: Quercetin contains anti-inflammatory qualities that may aid in the reduction of inflammation in the prostate gland and surrounding tissues. Chronic inflammation has been linked to a variety of prostate diseases.

3. Prostate Cancer: Some studies indicate that quercetin may have anti-cancer characteristics, and research into its possible function in preventing or reducing the growth of prostate cancer cells is ongoing. More research, however, is required to confirm its efficacy clearly.

4. urine Health: Quercetin may help relieve urine symptoms caused by benign prostatic hyperplasia (BPH), a non-cancerous enlargement of the prostate that can cause urinary issues.

5. Quercetin can be present in a range of foods, including apples, onions, citrus fruits, berries, red grapes, broccoli, and tea. A diet high in these foods may naturally supply you with quercetin.

6. Supplements: Quercetin supplements are available and may be used to boost quercetin consumption, especially if enough levels are difficult to obtain from dietary sources. However, before utilizing supplements, contact with a healthcare expert to ensure they are appropriate for your health needs.

While quercetin appears to be beneficial for prostate health, it is crucial to note that it should be part of a comprehensive healthy lifestyle that includes a balanced diet, frequent exercise, and proactive healthcare management. If you have specific concerns about your prostate health, such as prostate cancer or urinary symptoms, speak with a healthcare specialist who can provide individualized advice and recommendations based on your unique situation.

What happens after your prostate has been removed?

Men frequently claim that their penis has shriveled after having their prostate removed due to cancer. However, there is still hope after even after an aggressive prostate cancer.

If your prostate is removed, you will almost certainly lose your ability to ejaculate. There is a chance (depending on what you read) that you will be incontinent and/or impotent.

The penis size shortens after a few days of the surgery and normalize in length after a year.

Depending on how close my cancer was to the nerves that controlled erections, the pair, which wrap around the prostate like a hand cupping a peach could be saved, keep one side, or, God forbid, remove those nerves entirely. You should expect to recover 2 years following the surgery.

Following a prostatectomy, or surgical removal of the prostate gland, various changes and issues occur.

The particular consequences and modifications required are determined by the type of prostatectomy performed (e.g., radical prostatectomy, laparoscopic, robotic-assisted, or open surgery) as well as an individual's overall health and lifestyle. Here are some common changes and characteristics to anticipate following prostate removal:

1. Urinary Changes

Following surgery, many men develop transient urine incontinence. This means they may have trouble controlling their urine flow and may leak. Most men improve and regain urinary control with time. Kegel exercises, which strengthen the pelvic floor muscles, can help with healing.

Catheter: A catheter is frequently used to empty urine from the bladder soon following surgery. It may remain in place for a short time, generally a week or two, until urinary function returns to normal.

Slow Recovery: It may take many weeks or months to restore full urinary control, and some men may develop long-term problems, though this is rare.

2. Sexual Function

It is normal for men to develop transient or permanent erectile dysfunction after prostate removal. During surgery, nerve-sparing procedures can help preserve erectile function, but recovery differs from person to person. To treat ED, medications, vacuum erection devices, penile implants, and other therapies can be investigated.

3. Fertility issues

Because the prostate's principal function is in sperm generation, and sperm production continues in the testes, prostate removal has no effect on a man's capacity to father children. Fertility may be harmed if surgery is combined with other treatments that affect the testes.

4. Lifestyle and Diet

Some dietary adjustments may be suggested to improve general health and lower the likelihood of adverse effects such as bladder irritation or constipation.

A healthy lifestyle that includes regular exercise and a well-balanced diet can help with recuperation and general well-being.

5. Continued Care

Follow-up appointments with the healthcare practitioner are required on a regular basis to monitor recovery and handle any concerns that may occur.

PSA (prostate-specific antigen) levels are typically monitored as part of the post-surgery treatment plan to detect any potential return of prostate cancer.

6. Emotional and Psychological Impact

A prostate cancer diagnosis and treatment can have emotional and psychological consequences for individuals and their relationships.

Support from healthcare providers, counselors, or support groups might be beneficial in dealing with these difficulties.

7. Cancer Treatment Continued

If a prostatectomy was performed as part of the prostate cancer treatment, further therapies, such as radiation therapy or hormone therapy, may be indicated depending on the stage and severity of the cancer.

It's crucial to note that the symptoms and recuperation time following prostate removal can vary greatly between people. The surgical method, individual health, and the level of cancer involvement all play a part in deciding the outcomes.

One will probably be able to resume sexual activity after recuperating from surgery. After simple prostatectomy, you can still have an orgasm during sex, but you'll ejaculate very little or no semen. After radical prostatectomy, full recovery of erectile function may take as long as 18 months for some men. Open and honest communication with healthcare providers is essential for addressing concerns and building a specific post-surgery care plan.

www.ingramcontent.com/pod-product-compliance
Lightning Source LLC
Chambersburg PA
CBHW070808260726

48660CB00005B/1763